Foreword

Instead of following a fad diet, or relying on heuristic advice to get into the shape they want, I believe people should learn the science that makes their bodies into what they are, and then apply that knowledge to achieve their goals. I'm baffled at how much pseudo-science is promulgated regarding working out, health, and diets. The science itself is well-researched and often easier to understand than "bro-science" or the newest workout plan. My goal in writing this essay is to take that science and condense it into an easy-to-digest format that anyone can read and understand.

After several friends had great success getting into shape after reading this text, I have decided to publish it.

While many scientific articles are cited in this text, it's not written strictly as academic literature, and all opinions expressed within are my own. This is not meant to be medical advice, but is an introduction into the research world of health. Hopefully this text helps a lot of people understand and take their physical health more into their own hands.

The Science of Getting in Shape

Getting in shape is more straightforward than you think. Most people view getting in shape as an amorphous black-box. You pay your dues to the pagan gods of abdominal muscles by going to the gym and eating salads, who in turn may either bless you with the body of your dreams, or arbitrarily refuse your burnt calorie offering. In reality, the entire process can be mathematically modeled, and if you know and satisfy the correct variables you can turn your body into whatever you want (within reason). In this essay, I will go through the science behind getting in shape, cite many studies conducted by physiatrists and athletic training researchers, and present the under-the-hood mathematical view of working out that pop-culture has concluded taboo.

You're not *that* Special

Everyone thinks that when it comes putting on muscle, losing weight, or metabolizing carbs, their body is an anomaly. The cosmopolitan bikini is unattainable, the fat rolls are an inherent part of your chi, and Dwayne the Rock Johnson is an urban myth. Most of the arguments I've heard boil down to the following categories:

"I just have a really low metabolism."

"I'm genetically fat."

"No matter how little I eat or how much I workout my weight never changes."

Everybody's bodies are different, and a very small fraction of people have strange diseases that affect their metabolism (much smaller than the fraction of people that claim to); but, nobody is above the laws of physics. The first law of thermodynamics is: *Energy can neither be created nor destroyed, but it can be changed from one form to another.* In other words, your body **does not** move without using energy, and that energy came from somewhere. Vice versa, you don't consume energy and then pee it out. You burn it. That's right, calories are a measure of *energy.* 1 calorie = 4.184 Joules of energy. A double-A battery typically contains about 10,000 Joules or 10,000/4.184 = 2390 calories. A gallon of gasoline may contain about 31,000 calories. You put gas in a car, the car moves, and the car burns calories, just like you. Every calorie that you eat or burn is accounted for by the first law of thermodynamics.

The Great Weight Equation

Let's build a full model to determine daily weight gain.

Calorie/Weight Conversion

Many scientists have spent a lot of time and money figuring out exactly how many calories are in a pound of fat and the answer is roughly 3,500 calories[50]. If you burn 3,500 more calories than you eat, you will lose a pound. If you eat 3,500 more calories than you burn, you will gain a pound. This gives us our first basic equation:

Pounds Gained Today = 3,500 * (Calories Eaten - Calories Burned)

Our body is generally accepted to both store and burn calories with impressive efficiency, so for our purposes this same equation can be used for both weight gain or weight loss.

Metabolism

Let's increase the measurability of this equation by adding in the different ways that calories are burned.

Calories burned = BMR + Exercise

The BMR (Basal Metabolic Rate) is the amount of calories you burn by simply existing. Your body requires calories to keep your brain functioning, replenish dying cells, fix itself, keep your blood pumping, and many other things.

Although the standard way to truly measure your metabolic rate is to hook you up to an oxygen monitor for 24 hours, recent scientific literature gives us a lot of ways to reasonably predict your metabolic rate. For a white premenopausal female, the best modeled equation is linear, and looks like this:

$$BMR = 301 + 10.2W + 3.09H - 3.09A[1]$$

Where W is weight in kilograms, H is height in centimeters, and A is age years. So if you are 5'9", weight 130 pounds, and are 22 years old current literature would predict your basal metabolic rate to be around 1376 calories / day. This means that if you didn't do anything and laid in bed all day you would burn 1376 calories / day. If you didn't work out and ate 2000 calories/day, you would likely gain a little over a pound every week.

Equations vary somewhat by demographic, and you can find the best-fit equation for your demographic in the literature review conducted by Sabounchi et. Al. in 2013[1] (the first citation at the end of this essay). There are outliers of some people that have higher metabolisms or lower metabolisms than others, and this basal metabolic rate metabolism equation models the average person. It should be noted that the standard deviation of metabolism by the weight coefficient is 15.2%[1]. While this equation would predict that that our hypothetical 22 year old female has a basal metabolic rate of 1376 calories, in reality her metabolic rate to one standard deviation is most likely somewhere between 1169.6 (on the lower end) and 1582.4 (on the higher end). This also means that about 1% of people in this age group will have a basal metabolic rate under 1000 calories/day, and 1% of people will have a basal metabolic rate above 1750 calories/day. It is *extremely* unlikely that your BMR is more than 30% different than the average person.

How to change your BMR

For the most part changing your basal metabolic rate isn't an option. You will require less and less calories as you age to keep your current weight. There is some variability to your metabolism that is accounted for by the standard deviation of the coefficients in the above equation.

The ways that you can increase your basal metabolic rate to put you on the higher end of that spectrum are:

1. Have more muscle than fat. Many studies show that maintaining muscle weight requires significantly more caloric expenditure than maintaining fat weight[51].

2. Mental stimulation. Creative thinking burns calories, about 20% of the average person's caloric intake goes to power their brain, and in some instances it

can be much higher than that. A Stanford professor claims grandmasters at chess tournaments to be burning 5000 calories daily and postulates that it is due to the high level of cognition.[52]

This BMR equation also explains how so many people trying to lose weight hit a "plateau" where their progress is stymied. As you lose weight your body requires less calories to maintain its new and smaller stature, and therefore the caloric intake that previously allowed you to lose half a pound a week becomes the caloric intake that maintains your current weight. Conversely, this leads to a similar plateau in individuals who are trying to gain weight. As you gain weight, your basal metabolic rate increases, so the same amount of food you needed to eat to go from 130-160lbs is not the same amount of food you need to eat to go from 160-190lbs.

Macronutrients

"It is crudely true that if a man's calorie intake is sufficient, he will somehow stagger to maturity, and he will reproduce" -Alfred Crosby.[2] The same cannot be said for any other nutritional measurement.

The most important number in your diet is the calorie. The most important nutritional metric in your food is the calorie. You can eat no sugar and still get fat, you can eat only sugar and still lose weight. You can eat all of the omega-3 fatty acids in the world and still die of malnutrition. Calories are a measure of energy, and by the first law of thermodynamics, if you want to reach or stay at a certain size, this is the nutritional value that should most concern you.

While macronutrients aren't going to get you in shape if your caloric intake is egregiously misallocated, once you have your caloric intake in line, macronutrients become important.

I'll *very roughly* sum up the recent literature on macronutrients in one line:

Consume more protein. Consume less sugar.

Generally, the three macronutrients of note are Protein, Fat, and Carbohydrate (sugar). Almost all of the calories that you eat are consumed in the form of these three macronutrients. While your weight is a function of the calories you consume, the form that those calories come in can change what that weight looks like, whether that weight is muscle/fat, and is important to your all around health.

Protein and Muscle

Proteins are the building blocks of your body. Fats are a store of energy. And Sugar is energy ready to be released at a moment's notice. It is impossible to gain muscle from a diet comprised mostly of sugar or even of fat because your body cannot build the necessary amino acids to create muscle[3] from sugar and fat. Fat cannot be turned into muscle. Sugar cannot be turned into muscle. They are chemically different. Sugar is made up of glycan rings, also known as sacharrides, that can easily be broken and metabolized in the presence of the right catalases, and fats are long chains of carbon that can be reduced as ketones (this is where the name for the keto diet comes from). Proteins are amino acids, which are what your body uses to build and replenish almost every part of itself. No matter how hard you work out, fat cannot be turned into muscle. Fat isn't built from amino acids, and muscle isn't built from fats. If you have fat and you want muscle, you need to burn the fat (metabolize through ketones) and build the muscle with protein.

When your body is at a calorie surplus, it will begin to add on weight. If you don't give it a reason to need muscle (ie. Working out), your body will not build muscle. If you don't give it proteins to use to build muscles, your body will not build muscle. If you want to gain weight and muscle you need to do 3 things:

1. Work out and give your body a reason to build more muscle.

2. Eat at a caloric surplus so that your body doesn't need to burn the protein for fuel and you can gain weight.

3. Consume enough protein that your body has amino acids to build muscle with instead of simply using the protein you have consumed to repair itself.

Most people in America do not eat enough protein and do their physique a great deal of disservice. Your body may be trying to build muscles, but is unable to do so for lack of amino acid building blocks. Many people in the United States would see less fat and more muscle on their bodies if they increased their protein intake and allowed their bodies to build what they are naturally trying to do. Recent scientific literature recommends 1.6g protein / kg of body weight (0.72g/lb) daily for active people[3]. For example, if you weigh 130 pounds and work out, you should be consuming 93.6g protein daily for your body to develop how it would like to, and avoid putting on unnecessary fat. You can work out like crazy, see little progress, and still have more fat than is natural if you are not consuming enough protein simply because your body has nothing it can build muscle with. One of the most cited nutritional pieces of scientific literature written in 2016 concludes: "Therefore, adequate consumption of high-quality proteins from animal products (e.g., lean meat and milk) is essential for optimal growth, development, and health of humans".[3] While it is possible to overeat protein, for it to begin to cause metabolic discomfort people typically need to be consuming more than 2g/pound of body weight daily, which is almost never going to happen. Even if you reached a ridiculous level of protein overconsumption, some research suggests that your body can adapt to that intake level quickly and begin to thrive.[3]

Your body is able to burn protein as a fuel source. If your body needs to, it will burn the protein you have consumed and get 4 calories per gram of protein. This is why it's so important to eat at a calorie surplus if you're trying to gain large amounts of muscle. Your body will preferentially burn sugar and fat first saving proteins to use for buidling. Eat enough protein so that when your metabolism is finished supporting your daily activities, your body still has some protein building blocks left over for muscle building. If you are trying to both lose weight and gain muscle simultaneously, you won't gain as much muscle as you would during a bulk/ surplus; however, with enough protein in your diet losing weight and gaining muscle at the same time is possible given that you have fat to burn. If you work out and send the right signals for muscle hypertrophy, your body will preferentially burn the fat on your body to keep your metabolism running, and then use the protein you eat to build muscle (more on this later).

Sugar

No matter what your body goals are, gaining or losing weight, if you live in modern society you are likely consuming too much sugar.

While fitness influences tout the evils of processed sugars as opposed to natural sugars, the evidence to support their claims is relatively lacking.[4] Sugar isn't inherently bad for you, sugar is simply the most readily available source of energy for your body. Sugar is calories in their most available form, the carbohydrate. It is good for providing lots of fast calories, but certainly not for building muscle. Whether you get your sugar from a jolly-rancher or from bread, it will serve the same purpose to your body: *ready to use calories.* People drink gatorade because they think it's better for you than soda - it has the same amount of sugar. People drink lots of juice because they think natural sugar is better than artificial sugar - believe it or not the sugar in soda is often just as natural as the sugar in juice. Sugar is usually harvested from cane or corn, which are both very natural, and then put into soda. A glass of grape juice often has more sugar than a soda, and lemonade usually has more sugar than almost any other beverage.

For millions of years of our ancestors up until 100 years ago or so, starving to death was not uncommon. A ready-to-go form of calories that your body can easily burn for energy or turn into fat to survive a food-scarce winter was basically gold. In fact, it is proven that sugar consumption makes people (especially young women for some reason) significantly hungrier.[5] Sugar tastes good because it is caloric and our ancestors who starved to death in caves evolved to eat as much of it as they can, and to increase their stomach capacity and get hungrier whenever they were presented with it, because they almost never got sugar. Remember: "It is crudely true that if a man's calorie intake is sufficient, he will somehow stagger to maturity, and he will reproduce." Little did evolution know that in 2022 some people would be consuming 90% of their daily calories in carbohydrate. Caloric drinks are perhaps the largest culprit in the weight gain of our society. Calories that go straight into your blood stream that you don't even have to chew... Caloric drinks move through your digestive system so fast that they rarely even satiate any hunger. (If you are trying to gain weight, go ahead, drink some soda after a work-out, calories in drinks are the quickest way to gain weight).

Sugar is the easiest way to gain fat. The health problems from an overconsumption of sugar are endless: Diabetes, obesity, kidney issues, liver issues, pulmonary issues, cognitive issues just to name a few. This is particularly concerning when drinking a single soda beverage or a glass of juice can be more sugar than one's entire recommended daily intake. While eating some sugar is part of a healthy diet, rare is the American who could not stand to gain from less sugar consumption.

Fats

Fats got a bad rap in the 90s, but now you've heard enough people say that fats "have a bad rap" that I don't think they really have a bad rap anymore. Fats are simply the most dense form of calories that you can eat. 9 calories / gram. Fats are very high in calories, so you can gain weight quickly by eating a lot of them; however, in our society they aren't as culpable sugar.

Fats are much harder to digest than sugar. Unlike sugar, fats don't quickly enter the blood stream and get turned into body fat. Often if fats are to be turned into body fat they first need to be turned into sugar through a process called gluconeogenesis, and then turned from sugar into body fat. Fats are much larger molecules than carbohydrates, and take much longer to digest. They will make you feel full for longer, improve brain function,[6] and taste great.

In my opinion, fats aren't something that you should be striving to eat a ton of; however, they certainly shouldn't be avoided, and heaven forbid they are replaced with sugar. Fats are a simply a dense source of energy that your body needs, and generally are going to keep you in better shape than getting those same calories from sugar.

I'll repeat myself:

Consume more protein. Consume less sugar.

Working out

Different people with different goals should work out in different ways; however, almost everybody should work out every day. Remember, Calories burned = BMR + *Exercise*.

Beginners Gains

When you first start working out, your body will adapt very quickly, and you will see what are known as "beginners gains." This is simply your body kicking into gear from being totally sedentary to restructuring itself to be ready to face some physical activity. After about 2 months to 10 weeks, the "beginners' gains" phase will start to wear off.[7] If you haven't been working out and begin working out every day, you will see very quick progress for the first couple of months almost no matter what you do. Whether your progress continues after that becomes very quickly dependent on the quality of your workout. This is why you will see people trying to lose weight that make a ton of progress in a few months, and then give up after they plateau at their beginner gains. This is also why you will see a guy who starts working out go from benching nothing to 165 in a couple of months, and then stay at that weight for the next two years. Beginners' gains come from working out however you do it at the beginning, but getting past the beginners' gains point requires working out in a way that makes more scientific sense.

Working out to Gain Muscle

First, do not be trying to gain muscle if you aren't eating enough protein. If you break down your muscles and there is nothing to build them back with, you can get weaker from working out.

Second, gaining muscle can be reduced to another equation!

Given that neither your protein intake nor your caloric intake are a limiting factor:

Muscle mass gained = Time your muscle spends rebuilding itself * the average speed at which your muscle rebuilds itself

This equation gives us two broadly-defined variables that we can work with to gain muscle:

Time your muscle spends rebuilding itself, and the average speed at which it rebuilds itself.

For muscle to spend time rebuilding itself, we need to break that muscle down. This is done by lifting weights, running, using machines, and working out. Muscle cells are made of fibers called sarcomeres which contain actin and myosin filaments. As the muscle is strained, these filaments pull together to contract the muscle. As the muscle is pushed to its limit, these filaments tear on a microscopic level. Blood rushes to the site of the tear carrying the nutrients necessary (proteins that you better be eating) to begin repairing the torn filaments giving the muscle a swollen look known to gym bros as "the pump." Your body is programmed to adapt, and when your muscles are getting shredded by your workout, your body will build them back up stronger such that they can handle the same workout without tearing.

If you want your muscles to grow for maximum size, the micro-tears need to be large and significant (not broken though, please don't tear your bicep). The first step to getting your muscles to spend a lot of time rebuilding themselves is to workout with heavy weights and few reps. The heavier the weights, the more significant the tears will be. Lots of small contractions do not break the muscle down in the same way a couple of massive contractions do. Think of it like a trampoline. Your 30 pound nephew jumping all day might tire him out, but you're not worried about the trampoline tearing at all until your 350 pound uncle gets on and does three cannonball bounces. Study after study after study has shown that high-weight exercise is lightyears ahead at creating muscle hypertrophy (breakdown, tears, and swelling) than light-weight high-rep exercise.[8] Studies across almost all exercises seem to show that sets in the vicinity of 8-12 reps maximizes hypertrophy for men. You might consider taking creatine which has been shown to increase the weight you can handle getting 8 reps with, which can increase the workout-hypertrophy.[15]

The scientific jury is still out on how many sets you should do when you train a muscle to maximize muscle mass and strength; however, several studies suggest that it is whatever gets you to at least 20 total reps. For example, if you are doing sets of 8, three sets would be sufficient.[11]

So if doing eight reps three times at a very heavy weight that will push you to failure on an exercise will break the muscle down maximally, how often should you workout each muscle? This comes down to the second part of our equation, maximizing the speed at which your muscle rebuilds:

Muscle growth is the highest 24 hours after a workout.[10] Don't believe the "you must drink protein right after the workout to maximize muscle growth" hype. You need to have a high daily protein consumption every day, because your muscle will grow back for the next 5-7 days, and it won't even reach its peak growth speed until 24 hours after your workout. Your body needs time to get nutrients to the site of the injury, and to set up regrowth. It doesn't happen instantaneously. Think of the trampoline analogy, after the trampoline is torn by your 350lb uncle's cannonball, the initial trauma needs to be assessed, and repairs won't be in full swing until tomorrow.

Okay, so if it takes 5-7 days for a muscle to regrow, does it help or hurt me to workout too often? Short answer is - it doesn't make very much of a difference. In a study comparing many different frequencies of heavyweight exercise on muscle growth done in 2018, the difference in muscle growth between working out the same muscle 1 time a week and 4 times a week was almost nothing.

"Difference in magnitude of effect between frequencies of 1 and 3+ days per week was modest. In conclusion, there is strong evidence that resistance training frequency does not significantly or meaningfully impact muscle hypertrophy when volume is equated. Thus, for a given training volume, individuals can choose a weekly frequency per muscle groups based on personal preference."[9]

To maximize growth make sure that you work out every muscle at least once a week. The athlete with a good diet that only works out each muscle once a week will very quickly overtake the athlete that has a poor diet and works every muscle daily spending 7 hours a day in the gym. If you are working out each muscle less than once a week, then you are certainly leaving gains on the table.

The other thing that can be done to increase the speed at which muscles grow and regenerate can be done by supplementation. While testosterone (steroids) and SARMs will increase the baseline regeneration speed, citruline-malate can decrease muscle recovery time by as much as 33%, allowing you to benefit significantly from working out the same muscle multiple times per week;[12] however, citruline-malate advantages are insignificant in untrained subjects.[13] Citruline is a precursor in your body to Arginine, which is one of the major building blocks of muscle, and attaching it to malic acid (malate) is postulated to allow it to pass through your system faster.

Working out to Lose Weight

If you are working out to lose weight, everything is going to come back to the great weight gain equation. Whatever you do to workout should be helping you to create and maintain a caloric deficit, which will cause you to lose weight.

While lifting weights will help build muscle which will increase your metabolism, many people trying to lose weight workout at the gym like they are trying to gain weight. High-rep low-frequency doesn't burn a lot of calories, and it helps your body put on more muscle. While I would recommend working out with heavy weights especially to maintain and build your larger and more important muscles for stability, core, glutes etc., your biceps are a very small percentage of your bodyweight, and focusing on biceps will not maximize weight loss. Even if you are working out for your muscles to stand-out, a smaller bicep with lower body fat on it looks much more impressive than a large bicep with a high fat-mass. It has been shown that strength training does not alter the fat around your muscles at all.[17] If you don't believe that watch a strongman competition.

To lose weight you should be primarily engaging in activities that burn calories. Calories burned from an exercise can be very easily calculated and visualized:

Calories are a measurement of energy. "Work" is a physics term used to measure energy required to do a specific task. Work is defined mathematically as "force times distance." Let's use the example of running. How much force it takes to move you depends on how much you weigh. You calculate the force required to move your weight in newtons, and then you multiply the distance you moved and you will get the energy required in joules, which can be readily converted into calories. Different models will predict different amounts of calories burned, but at 130 pounds you will burn about 90 calories per mile moved.[14] While different speeds and walking/running involve various mechanics, simplifying the amount of calories burned running to a Force*Distance work equation will be more accurate than trying to measure calories burned as a measure of time. The faster you run the more calories you will burn every minute, because you are doing more "work" pushing the your weight across a greater distance.

In my opinion, losing weight by eating significantly fewer calories than you burn while remaining sedentary is a difficult way to lose weight. It requires a lot of self-control, and isn't nearly as satisfying. Losing weight by working out has additional benefits, cardio, muscle tone, and doesn't require nearly as much of a cutback on caloric intake (please make sure you're eating enough protein though).

Let's do the math:

Lets say you weigh 150 pounds and you want to get down to 130. If we round your calories burned/mile to 100 calories, you need to run 5 miles a day to lose a pound per week (remember one pound is 3500 calories, 7 * 500 = 3500). Provided you eat at your normal metabolic rate, if you run 5 miles/day for 5 months, you will lose the weight.

One problem I have seen in a lot of people that are trying to lose weight is that they don't run very far because they can't run very far. While our ancestors would trek 20 miles per day to keep up with the mammoth herds, some of us haven't run or walked very much in years, and have gotten to the point where we can barely run or walk one or two miles at a time. If you only run one mile a day, you will only be burning around 100 calories a day. At that pace it will take 3 years to lose 20 pounds, or more likely, be insignificant. The great thing about the physics work equation is that it doesn't matter how long it takes you to cover a distance, the work is the same. If you can only run one mile a day to start, I would suggest walking the other four until you can run two miles and walk three, and eventually you will get there. If you are running at a 7 minute mile pace, which more people than you think can achieve after running for a few months, running 5 miles will only take 35 minutes, and you'll have burned 500 calories.

Do I need to Lose Weight?

The internet will tell you no, and that you can be healthy at any weight. The heart that loves everybody might want to say no because it hurts to confront truth. But if you are overweight your real heart struggling to pump blood through more body than it was designed for will scream at you: yes. The millions of obese people that die in their 50s every year will scream at you: yes.

On the flip-side, it is extremely important to not lose more weight than you should. The reason your body puts on fat in the first place is to keep you from falling underweight. Thousands of bulimic and anorexic people die every year thinking they are overweight when in fact their underweight stature is literally killing them. Being underweight presents with health problems just as severe as obesity, including mental fog, lack of energy, and injury-prone bones.

Everybody should strive to maintain both a healthy weight, and a healthy physique. Don't be overweight, don't be underweight, and if you are a good weight, your body will feel better and you will live longer if you have good cardio and healthy muscle mass.

BMI

Recently there has been a lot of hate for BMI (Body Mass Index). BMI is still the standard way to define overweight and underweight in medicine, and your primary care physician will still likely use it to determine whether you should try to lose weight. It's a very simple formula: Weight in Kg / Height in M squared. Below 18.5 is underweight, above 25 is overweight, and above 30 is obese. The range from 18.5 to 25 is a fairly broad range that can fit a lot of different body types, all of which are concerned medically not underweight nor overweight.

Lets say you are 5'8", anywhere from ~122 pounds to ~160 pounds is considered a normal weight. If you are under 122 pounds you should in general consider lifting weights and eating more, if you are approaching 160 pounds you should in general consider increasing your calories burned through cardio and decreasing caloric intake.

Many people recently have criticized the BMI as too rudimentary and not accounting for fringe cases; however, I think that the BMI includes a surprisingly diverse group of bodies. I have heard on many occasions that BMI is a bad measurement because it would consider Lebron James as overweight. Lebron has a BMI of 26.8, which would indeed put him as overweight, and yes, Lebron is in phenomenal shape. Lebron, however, spends millions of dollars every year on his body to make sure that he can maintain that extra weight in a healthy way, including personal chefs for every meal, many doctors and professional nutritionists, and works out up to eight hours a day. I will suggest a BMI addendum to account for almost all of these fringe cases: if you can a. Run a mile in under 6 minutes, and b. Look like a greek god, don't worry about your BMI putting you in the overweight category. If you are in the overweight category because you have hulking muscle reserves and no body fat, I trust you know who you are. Otherwise, listen to your BMI. On the flip side, if you have a BMI of 17 please please please don't lose anymore weight, you're scientifically underweight, NOT fat, and you should start increasing your caloric intake or you could suffer health consequences.

Working out to Stay in Shape

Let's say that you are in great shape, no, you don't get to eat whatever you want now and never workout again. It is easier to maintain good health than it is create it or get back to it; but, it still requires work.

Maintaining your Weight

Again, maintaining your weight goes back to the great weight equation. Make sure you are eating the same amount of calories that you are burning, and you will maintain your weight. If you have been running to get into a certain shape, and you have lost the weight you needed to lose, I would suggest eating more to maintain weight rather than giving up running.

Maintaining your Muscle

Make sure you are eating enough to not lose weight, and make sure you are eating enough protein to be able to replenish muscle consistently. To maintain your muscle mass you don't need to work out as frequently as you did while you were gaining it; however, your muscle strength begins to deteriorate as soon as two-three weeks without working out according to a study published in *Sports Med*.[16]

Maintaining your Cardio

Make sure you keep getting cardiovascular exercise. Heart problems are one of the leading causes of death in the United States, and if you don't use it you lose it. Make sure that you are getting your heart rate up for an extended period of time several times a week minimum. This can be through running, intense weight-lifting, or playing sports (my favorite option).

Which Exercises are the Best

Believe it or not, between all of the bro-science, there is a lot of scientific literature about different exercises, and which exercises perform the best.

Reps Sets and Intensity

As cited above, to maximize muscle growth, you generally want to do about 8 reps per set, fail somewhere between the eighth and twelfth rep, and do 3 sets. This is true for almost all muscles. Don't believe the hype that doing 200 sit-ups is going to give you massive abs. Your abs are made of the same sarcomeres that your chest is made of, you need something more intense that you can't do 200 times. Think of the nephew on the trampoline.

There are a couple of exceptions to this Rep/Sets rule.

1. If you are female. Women have better responses and gains with lighter weight and higher repetition than men. Well this has been debated on the scientific field, one of the leading theories is that estrogen changes their glucose uptake process. If you are a woman, instead of doing sets that max you out at 8 reps, you might get better results from doing lighter weight sets with maxing out at 15-25 reps per set.

2. If you are training for endurance/tone rather than bulk. By far the most important factor in how toned your muscles look is body fat %. Small muscles can look extremely toned if there is no fat on them or in them. There are two different types of muscles in your body, slow-twitch and fast-twitch muscles. They are distinguished based on their preference for slow aerobic exercise burning lots of oxygen making them look red, vs fast single-rep force that doesn't use as much oxygen and burns out faster.

Build aerobic muscles for the "toned runner look" by using low weight high repetition, build fast-twitch muscles for huge bulk and one-rep strength to look like Dwayne the Rock Johnson.

Chest

Nothing beats the tried and true free-weight bench press for building pectoral mass.[18]

Biceps

Use a bar for your curls. Both undulated bars ($p<0.001$) and straight barbells have been conclusively shown to isolate the bicep more effectively than dumbbells.[19]

Triceps

The exercise that most activates the triceps is the triangle pushup while dips are a close second and kickbacks are the best activating weighted exercise.[21] Use a combination of these exercises when working on tricep growth depending on your goals. While the triangle pushup gives the best activation, it is the hardest to vary weight. Close-grip bench press is a secondary tricep exercise at best.

Deltoids

Lateral raises and shoulder presses are the best exercises. For the anterior deltoid the exercise that best activates the muscle is the shoulder press, and for all other parts of the deltoid muscle the lateral raise is much more effective. Lateral raises with dumbells more than double the deltoid EEG activation of shoulder benches or shoulder presses.[20] Incline bench isn't nearly as effective as shoulder press and lateral raises in shoulder activation.

Abdominals

Leg raises seem to be the most effective exercise for stimulating the rectus abdominis (the six-pack area), while other exercises are necessary to effectively stimulate the oblique abdominals.[22] Many commercial machines have been shown to activate the abdominals more effectively than body-weight exercises. Of note is the "Ab Slide."[23] Overall, leg-raises are some of the most effective abdominally stimulating exercises. Crunches and sit-ups are not as effective. While machines rarely are shown to be more effective than free-weights and barbells, for abdominal exercises machines can help create an otherwise impossible weighted scenario to help get the user to be able to get into the 8-12 rep sweet-spot for their torso.

While many people do abdominal exercises to lose fat around their midriff, it should be noted that training your abdominals will not result in a loss of midriff fat, it will simply result in stronger abdominals. This question was answered in a 2011 study.[24] To "get a 6-pack," reducing your body-fat percentage is key. Building your abdominal muscles may make them more visible, but the layer of fat must be removed if you want a visible 6-pack.

Latissimus Dorsi

Inverted rows are the best for stimulating the medial latissimus dorsi as measured via EMG, but other exercises involving trunk rotation are shown to be more effective in stimulating the lateral parts of the muscle.[28] The latissimus dorsi is one of the largest muscles in the body, and it's worth doing different exercises to stimulate it. The lat-pull is also extremely effective, and one study suggests that using a V-shaped bar shows the best EMG activity.[29] Consider using a V-shaped bar for your pull-ups or lat pull-downs.

The Glutes

Are an often over-looked muscle-group.

Your gluteal muscles are responsible for controlling the most important joint for improving your vertical.[31]

One study showed training glutes increases jump-height an average of 17.15% in 8 weeks.[32]

Trainers online tend to agree that the glutes are the most important muscles to the vertical jump,[33] which makes sense considering that they are the largest muscle in the body.

[The Gluteus Maximus] was likely evolved for the purpose of running unlike any other primate.[34]

[The Gluteus Maximus exists for] stabilizing the body and preventing injury and pain while running.[35]

If you want to jump higher, run faster, or have less pain and get injured less, make sure to train your glutes.

Several studies have shown the muscle activation of different exercises for the glutes. The step-up across multiple studies has been shown to be the most effective exercise, do it holding free-weights to get to a desired power level.

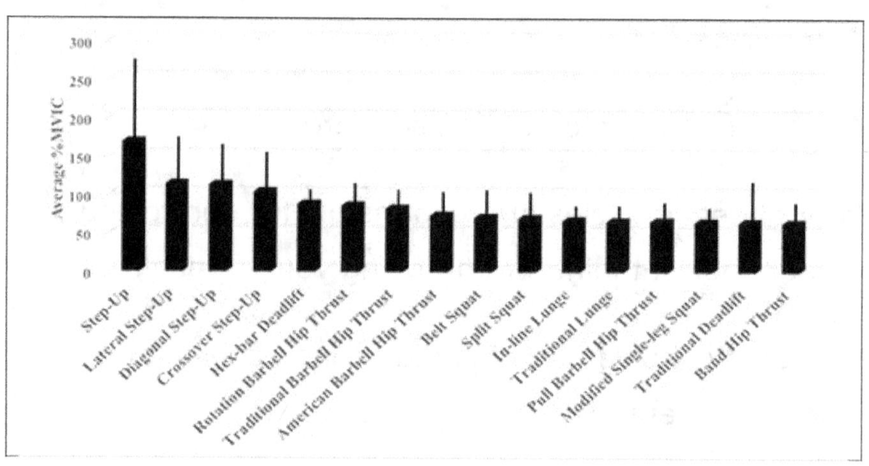

Figure: (Neto 2020)[36]

Out of bodyweight exercises the plank with hip-extension rankedsurprisingly high, MVIC=106.[37]

Deadlifts and squats are also effective at targeting the glutes, and are also found as top exercises for many other lower-body muscles. The hex-bar deadlifts seem to be the most effective for targeting the glutes themselves, but there is some conflicting information on this as Romanian deadlifts and normal deadlifts are shown to be extremely effective (up to MVIC=94) in some studies.[38]

Whatever your getting-in-shape goals, make sure that you have a regimen to keep your glutes activated consistently. As the biggest muscle in the body, if you want to decrease body-fat percentage quickly, increasing the size of the glutes is the most effective single-muscle group target.

Hamstrings

Hamstrings are important for sprinting speed. If you want to run quickly, your hamstrings need to be able to contract with a lot of force. The most effective exercise for hamstring strength is hands-down the Romanian deadlift.[39] Other unconventional exercises such as the Russian curl can also be effective.

Quadriceps

Representing 4 different muscles in the anterior chamber of the thigh, the quadriceps are an important leg muscle for stability, vertical jump, and "bounce" while running. A 2019 study suggests that all squat variations activate the quadriceps similarly.[40] Workout forums seem to suggest that the front-squat is more effective in quad stimulation. Make sure that you do squats to complete a lower-body exercise.

Gastrocnemius/Soleus

Out of just the leg muscles, the lateral gastrocnemius thickness is the strongest predictor of jumping ability.[30] Weighted calf-raises are the exercise of choice to train your calves, and out of their variations "one can chose between exercises based on personal preferences and practical aspects, without any negative impact on muscle activation."[41]

Machines vs Bodyweight vs Free-weight

One area that divides the fitness community is whether to train with machines, bodyweight, or using free-weights. Let's go over some of the comparisons:

Because it is important to stay within an optimal repetition range, exercises that involve the bodyweight only will lead to strength plateaus. Not a lot of research has been done to compare full body-weight regimens to free-weight only regimens; however, one such study in 2018 with female test-subjects had one group train with bodyweight and the other with free weights. At the end of 8 weeks they were unable to prove any increase in strength whatsoever from the bodyweight group, while they found significant increase in strength in the free-weight group.[49]

Machines allow the user to adjust the weight, and keep a steady amount of weight throughout the exercise. Pure muscle mass can be achieved almost equally using either machines or free-weight.[42] Training with free-weights seems to provide several advantages over machines:

Instability of the free-weights allows the user to maintain a level of inhibitory control.[43]

Training with free-weights is connected to higher testosterone levels in men.[44]

Free-weight training may afford the user greater perception which may help avoid injuries.[53]

Training with free-weights provides advantages over the other options with few drawbacks.

Workout Plans

Here are some example workout plans by goal and body type:

Looking to gain weight and muscle mass:

Designed to give each muscle maximum stimulus, and work any muscle two days in a row.

Diet: 500 - 750 daily calorie surplus. 1g protein + /lb.

Day 1 (shoulder girdle): Bench Press. Lateral Raises. Shoulder Press. Leg Raises/ ab machine (abs).

Day 2 (Arms/Back): Barbell curls. Tricep kickbacks. V-bar Lat pulls. Inverted rows.

Day 3 (legs): weighted step-ups. Trap-bar deadlifts. Romanian Deadlifts. Front-squats. Obliques (ab machine).

Do these workouts once a week, or twice a week, depending on caloric intake, time available, and supplement use (creatine/citruline).

Looking to improve vertical jump:

Same as weight gain and muscle mass except another day is added between days 1 and 2 (the exercises from day 1.5 can also be mixed into days 1-3 to increase workout length)

Day 1.5 (vertical): Weighted calf-raises. Heavy back squats. Box-jumps. Running high-jumps split by leg. Normal Deadlifts. Cleans.

Looking to increase general athleticism:

Diet: No calorie deficit, error on the side of surplus, 1g protein/lb.

Day 1 (Increase speed muscles): 4x400 sprints. Romanian Deadlift. Weighted Calf Raises. Front squats.

Day 2 (Increase distance muscles): 5 mile run (or equivalent other exercise).

Day 3 (vertical): see day 1.5 in vertical jump.

Day 4 (shoulder girdle): see Day 1 to gain weight and muscle mass

Day 5 (Arms/Back): see Day 2 to gain weight and muscle mass

Repeat weekly and intersperse with sports/other athletic activity.

Male looking to lose weight and get an "instagram"-type body:

This is to lose weight, create visible abs, decrease the body fat % to accentuate angles in the face, increase upper body strength (pecs, biceps, triceps), and achieve a low body fat %. This will require to start with a deficit to lose weight, and involve a fair amount of weight-training and aerobic activity.

Diet: 500-1000 calorie deficit. 1g protein / lb.

5-mile run or equivalent EVERY DAY.

Do all three days of "gain weight and muscle mass" workout once/week to make sure that muscle mass increases WHILE weight is shed.

Once abs are visible around body-fat % of 8 or less, get rid of the calorie deficit but continue the workouts.

Female looking to lose weight and get an "instagram"-type body:

This is to lose weight, create visible abs, decrease the body fat % to accentuate angles in the face, firm the arms, and increase lower body strength (glutes, hamstrings, calves).

Diet 500-1000 calorie deficit. 0.8-1g protein / lb.

5-mile run or equivalent EVERY DAY.

Day 1 (glutes): Weighted step-ups. Hip thrusts. Hex-bar deadlifts.

Day 2 (arms/abs): Triangle pushups (or normal pushups until you can do triangle pushups). Leg raises. Ab-machine.

Day 3 (hamstrings/quads): 4x100 sprints. Romanian Deadlifts. Weighted front-squats. Weighted back-squats.

Day 4 (oblique sport): Play a sport that activates your obliques ie. Tennis, Soccer, swimming.

Do these four days once a week. There is no need to use weights every day, you really only need to use weights 3 times a week. There will be almost no benefit to using weights more than this. Losing weight from a calorie deficit and running every day will decrease body-fat percentage and these two items will be the most important for getting abs and a thin waist. Days 1 and 3 will tone and increase the muscles in the waist area significantly even while losing weight. Day 2 will make sure that there is muscle in the arms so that they are firm. Get rid of the calorie deficit once your BMI reaches your ideal level, be careful to not fall underweight. People are evolutionarily attracted to fitness and health, watch your BMI carefully as to not go underweight.

How long will it take to see results?

Regardless of your program of choice, take a measurement every week. Measure your BMI, Body Fat %, and repetition maxes to track your progress. You should be able to look in the mirror and see a marked difference in two months if you strictly adhere to one of the above programs. It will probably take about 6 months to reach an "instagram" goal, but once there it is easier to maintain.

500 calorie exercises (5 mile run equivalents):

This is a list of exercises that when done correctly will burn about 500 calories for the average person.

Run 5 miles

Walk 6 miles*

Swim 1 mile

Bike 20 miles

Hike 4 miles at a slight incline

Ultimate frisbee 1 hour

Golf walking w/ bag 2 hours

Basketball 1 hour

**Walking 6 miles burns a similar number of calories to running 5 miles. This does not contradict thermodynamics; cars burn more gas per mile going 100mph than going 45mph just like you burn more calories running a mile than walking a mile. Running is slightly less calorically efficient. There are many reasons for this, and the efficiency varies based on your running form (are you bouncing) and your muscular build (how much energy is coming from aerobic vs anaerobic processes).

Diet Plans

There is no single one-size-fits-all diet plan for people trying to gain muscle or lose weight. People have different taste preferences, diverse gut microbiota, and distinct religious/medical restrictions. After using the great weight equation, establishing a workout plan, reasonable fitness goals, and caloric goals, a diet plan will help you the rest of the way.

Hydration Caveat

Your weight will fluctuate as you drink water, sweat, eat, and void. Wrestlers take advantage of this, dropping unhealthy amounts of weight before matches. Although I won't cover hydration in detail in this text, if somebody is weighing themselves to monitor their health or progress, it is important to understand the following:

1. Do not become emotionally invested in rapid weight changes you see on the scale. Your weight will vary up to a couple of pounds daily, as you sweat, void, empty your bowels, eat, and drink. If you weight two pounds less in one day, it is unlikely that this is a permanent change. This is likely either dehydration or normal weight fluctuation. Weekly measurements are much more meaningful, and it will be difficult to discern the difference between normal weight fluctuation and loss of fat/gain of muscle until you've been measuring for a month.

2. You must stay hydrated. I've known people trying to lose weight who fell into this trap. If you stay dehydrated for an extended period of time you can keep your weight on the scale a pound or two lower than it should be. This is one of the reasons that weight itself is not a perfect measure of progress. While you might be able to weigh slightly less by keeping your body dehydrated, typically this does not transfer to an improved aesthetic result. Dehydration causes a host of unsavory health problems that I won't cover in this text, and is not an aesthetically appealing look. If you are trying to lose weight, do not cheat by dehydrating yourself. Don't kid yourself — "dehydrated and overweight" is not preferable to simply "overweight."

Psychology of Weight-Loss

Many people can adhere to a diet for a few months, but then get tired of it or "cheat" and quickly regress to where they were previously. Any changes you make you must be willing to make as permanent changes. Diets or workouts that you are only planning on using to get you to a certain weight will obviously not be effective long-term.

Changing only diet or only workout activity is at least 20% less effective than changing both, and changing only diet has a significant relapse rate. This is proposed to be mainly a psychological mechanism.[46]

Getting in shape provides a huge amount of psychological benefits. While it is possible to feel good about oneself without being in shape, weight loss is empirically shown to increase self-esteem, mitigate depression, and help a host of psychological issues in both genders, but this is especially pronounced in women.[47,48] The benefits of getting into shape are many, and you will be happier for many reasons, but that's beyond the scope of this paper.

Psychological challenges might make it harder to stay in shape, but the health-consequences of an inactive lifestyle remain just as severe (although the consequences themselves are not within the scope of this paper).

Injury and Pain Prevention

There are benefits to certain exercises to prevent pain.

It used to be thought that heavy deadlifting would cause back pain because of the extra strain put on the back. The research has recently concluded that the opposite is true.[45] People who incorporated deadlifts into their exercises consistently had significantly less low back pain. Even people with low back pain that began deadlifting had less low back pain. Strain on the spine is hypothesized to cause lower back pain, and deadlifting increases lower back strength, and the muscles in the back are able to bear a lot of the burden instead of the spine.

Conclusion

You're not above the laws of thermodynamics. It is possible for you to get into shape. You may have psychological challenges that make it difficult, but most likely you just need a little guidance on how to do it. When you make changes, make sure that you are willing to make them permanently. Don't do anything that you won't be able to do forever. Understand the science, commit, and you will see results. Follow the science, and if you don't "cheat" the science proves that you will see results.

Afterword

Much of getting in shape is a hotly debated topic, and many people hold zealous views regarding their current workout plan or trend. As I have been writing this and discussing workout concepts with friends, I've noticed how many people are willing to die on a hill for their workout beliefs. I'm not sure what it is about health science that seems to religiously separate people into schools of thought, but we should always stay open to new information.

As more information is discovered there may be more versions of this essay written, and some current scientific studies may be proven wrong. Stay up to date with the literature, and always be open to learning more! If you believe that certain parts of this essay are incorrect, or outdated takes on the science, please send me an email. *medicalschoolresearcher@gmail.com*

Citations

1. Sabounchi NS, Rahmandad H, Ammerman A. Best-fitting prediction equations for basal metabolic rate: informing obesity interventions in diverse populations. Int J Obes (Lond). 2013 Oct;37(10):1364-70. doi: 10.1038/ijo.2012.218. Epub 2013 Jan 15. PMID: 23318720; PMCID: PMC4278349. Retrieved from https://www.ncbi.nlm.nih.gov/pmc/articles/PMC4278349/

2. Crosby, A. (n.d.). Retrieved from https://warwick.ac.uk/fac/arts/history/research/centres/foodhistory/the_columbian_exchange_biological_and_cultural_consequences_of_1492_----_5_new_world_foods_and_old_world_demography_.pdf

3. Wu, G. (2016). Dietary protein intake and human health. Food Funct., 7(3), 1251-1265. doi:10.1039/c5fo01530h

4. Stanhope, K. L. (2016). Sugar consumption, metabolic disease and obesity: The state of the controversy. Crit Rev Clin Lab Sci., 53(1), 52-67. doi:10.3109/10408363.2015.1084990

5. Penaforte, F. R., Japur, C. C., Pigatto, L. P., Chiarello, P. G., & Diez-Garcia, R. W. (2013). Short-term impact of sugar consumption on hunger and ad libitum food intake in young women. Nutr Res Pract., 7(2), 77-81. doi:10.4162/nrp.2013.7.2.77

6. Weinandy, L. (2018). https://wexnermedical.osu.edu/blog/boost-your-brain-power-with-the-right-nutrition

7. Willoughby, D. S., Stout, J. R., & Wilborn, C. D. (2007). Effects of resistance training and protein plus amino acid supplementation on muscle anabolism, mass, and strength. Amino Acids, 32(4), 467-477. doi:10.1007/s00726-006-0398-7

8. Schoenfeld, B. J., Peterson, M. D., Ogborn, D., Contreras, B., & Sonmez, G. T. (2015). Effects of low- vs. high-load resistance training on muscle strength and hypertrophy in well-trained men. J Strength Cond Res., 29(10), 2954-2963. doi:10.1519/JSC.0000000000000958

9. Schoenfeld, B. J., Grgic, J., & Krieger, J. (2019). How many times per week should a muscle be trained to maximize muscle hypertrophy? A systematic review and meta-analysis of studies

examining the effects of resistance training frequency. J Sports Sci., 37(11), 1286-1295. doi:10.1080/02640414.2018.1555906

10. MacDougall, J. D., Gibala, M. J., Tarnopolsky, M. A., MacDonald, J. R., Interisano, S. A., & Yarasheski, K. E. (1995). The time course for elevated muscle protein synthesis following heavy resistance exercise. Can J Appl Physiol., 20(4), 480-486. doi:10.1139/h95-038

11. Baz-Valle, E., Fontes-Villalba, M., & Santos-Concejero, J. (2021). Total number of sets as a training volume quantification method for muscle hypertrophy: A systematic review. Journal of Strength and Conditioning Research, 35(3), 870-878. doi:10.1519/JSC.0000000000002776

12. Pérez-Guisado, J., & Jakeman, P. M. (2010). Citrulline malate enhances athletic anaerobic performance and relieves muscle soreness. Journal of Strength and Conditioning Research, 24(5), 1215-1222. doi:10.1519/JSC.0b013e3181cb28e0

13. da Silva, D. K., Jacinto, J. L., de Andrade, W. B., Roveratti, M. C., Estoche, J. M., Balvedi, M. C. W., de Oliveira, D. B., da Silva, R. A., & Aguiar, A.

F. (2017). Citrulline malate does not improve muscle recovery after resistance exercise in untrained young adult men. Nutrients, 9(10), 1132. doi:10.3390/nu9101132

14. Calories. (n.d.). Retrieved from https://www.rungeni.com/calories-burned-running-calc/

15. Kreider, R. B. (2003). Effects of creatine supplementation on performance and training adaptations. Molecular and Cellular Biochemistry, 244(1-2), 89-94. doi:10.1023/A:1023470610231

16. McMaster, D. T., Gill, N., Cronin, J., & McGuigan, M. (2013). The development, retention and decay rates of strength and power in elite rugby union, rugby league and American football: a systematic review. Sports Medicine, 43(5), 367-384. doi:10.1007/s40279-013-0031-3

17. Walts, C. T., Hanson, E. D., Delmonico, M. J., Yao, L., Wang, M. Q., & Hurley, B. F. (2008). Do sex or race differences influence strength training effects on muscle or fat? Medicine and Science in Sports and Exercise, 40(4), 669-676. doi:10.1249/MSS.0b013e318161aa82

18. Ogasawara, R., Thiebaud, R. S., Loenneke, J. P., Loftin, M., & Abe, T. (2012). Time course for arm and chest muscle thickness changes following bench press training. Interventional Medicine and Applied Science, 4(4), 217-220. doi:10.1556/IMAS.4.2012.4.7

19. Marcolin, G., Panizzolo, F. A., Petrone, N., Moro, T., Grigoletto, D., Piccolo, D., & Paoli, A. (2018). Differences in electromyographic activity of biceps brachii and brachioradialis while performing three variants of curl. PeerJ, 6, e5165. doi:10.7717/peerj.5165

20. Campos, Y. A. C., Vianna, J. M., Guimarães, M. P., Oliveira, J. L. D., Hernández-Mosqueira, C., da Silva, S. F., & Marchetti, P. H. (2020). Different Shoulder Exercises Affect the Activation of Deltoid Portions in Resistance-Trained Individuals. Journal of Human Kinetics, 75, 5-14. https://doi.org/10.2478/hukin-2020-0033

21. Boehler, B. S., Porcari, J. P., Kline, D., Hendrix, C. R., & Foster, C. (2012). Ace terrific triceps. https://acewebcontent.azureedge.net/certifiednews/images/article/pdfs/ACETricepsStudy.pdf

22. Park, D. J., & Park, S. Y. (2019). Which trunk exercise most effectively activates abdominal muscles? A comparative study of plank and isometric bilateral leg raise exercises. Journal of Back and Musculoskeletal Rehabilitation, 32(5), 797-802. https://doi.org/10.3233/BMR-181122

23. Escamilla, R. F., McTaggart, M. S., Fricklas, E. J., DeWitt, R., Kelleher, P., Taylor, M. K., Hreljac, A., & Moorman, C. T. (2006). An electromyographic analysis of commercial and common abdominal exercises: implications for rehabilitation and training. Journal of Orthopaedic & Sports Physical Therapy, 36(2), 45-57. https://doi.org/10.2519/jospt.2006.36.2.45

24. Vispute, S. S., Smith, J. D., LeCheminant, J. D., & Hurley, K. S. (2011). The effect of abdominal exercise on abdominal fat. Journal of Strength and Conditioning Research, 25(9), 2559-2564. https://doi.org/10.1519/JSC.0b013e3181fb4a46

25. Park, S. Y., Yoo, W. G., An, D. H., Oh, J. S., Lee, J. H., & Choi, B. R. (2015). Comparison of isometric exercises for activating latissimus dorsi against the upper body weight. Journal of Electromyography and Kinesiology, 25(1), 47-52. https://doi.org/10.1016/j.jelekin.2014.09.001

26. Escamilla, R. F., McTaggart, M. S., Fricklas, E. J.,
DeWitt, R., Kelleher, P., Taylor, M. K., Hreljac, A.,
& Moorman, C. T. (2006). An electromyographic
analysis of commercial and common abdominal
exercises: implications for rehabilitation and
training. Journal of Orthopaedic & Sports
Physical Therapy, 36(2), 45-57. doi:10.2519/
jospt.2006.36.2.45

27. Vispute, S. S., Smith, J. D., LeCheminant, J. D.,
& Hurley, K. S. (2011). The effect of abdominal
exercise on abdominal fat. Journal of Strength
and Conditioning Research, 25(9), 2559-2564.
doi:10.1519/JSC.0b013e3181fb4a46

28. Park, S. Y., Yoo, W. G., An, D. H., Oh, J. S., Lee,
J. H., & Choi, B. R. (2015). Comparison of
isometric exercises for activating latissimus dorsi
against the upper body weight. Journal of
Electromyography and Kinesiology, 25(1), 47-52.
doi:10.1016/j.jelekin.2014.09.001

29. Sperandei, S., Barros, M. A., Silveira-Júnior, P.
C., & Oliveira, C. G. (2009). Electromyographic
analysis of three different types of lat pull-down.
Journal of Strength and Conditioning Research,
23(7), 2033-2038. doi:10.1519/
JSC.0b013e3181b8d30a

30. Earp, J. E., Joseph, M., Kraemer, W. J., Newton, R. U., Comstock, B. A., Fragala, M. S., Dunn-Lewis, C., Solomon-Hill, G., Penwell, Z. R., Powell, M. D., Volek, J. S., Denegar, C. R., Häkkinen, K., & Maresh, C. M. (2010). Lower-body muscle structure and its role in jump performance during squat, countermovement, and depth drop jumps. Journal of Strength and Conditioning Research, 24(3), 722-729. doi:10.1519/JSC.0b013e3181d32c04

31. Lees A, Vanrenterghem J, De Clercq D. The maximal and submaximal vertical jump: implications for strength and conditioning. J Strength Cond Res. 2004 Nov;18(4):787-91. doi: 10.1519/14093.1. PMID: 15574084.

32. Gallego-Izquierdo T, Vidal-Aragón G, Calderón-Corrales P, Acuña Á, Achalandabaso-Ochoa A, Aibar-Almazán A, Martínez-Amat A, Pecos-Martín D. Effects of a Gluteal Muscles Specific Exercise Program on the Vertical Jump. Int J Environ Res Public Health. 2020 Jul 27;17(15):5383. doi: 10.3390/ijerph17155383. PMID: 32726899; PMCID: PMC7432749.

33. Harvey. 2022. Jump Stronger. https://jumpstronger.com/most-important-muscles-vertical-jump/

34. Lieberman DE, Raichlen DA, Pontzer H, Bramble DM, Cutright-Smith E. The human gluteus maximus and its role in running. J Exp Biol. 2006 Jun;209(Pt 11):2143-55. doi: 10.1242/jeb.02255. PMID: 16709916.

35. Semciw A, Neate R, Pizzari T. Running related gluteus medius function in health and injury: A systematic review with meta-analysis. J Electromyogr Kinesiol. 2016 Oct;30:98-110. doi: 10.1016/j.jelekin.2016.06.005. Epub 2016 Jun 17. PMID: 27367574.

36. Neto WK, Soares EG, Vieira TL, Aguiar R, Chola TA, Sampaio VL, Gama EF. Gluteus Maximus Activation during Common Strength and Hypertrophy Exercises: A Systematic Review. J Sports Sci Med. 2020 Feb 24;19(1):195-203. PMID: 32132843; PMCID: PMC7039033.

37. Boren K, Conrey C, Le Coguic J, Paprocki L, Voight M, Robinson TK. Electromyographic analysis of gluteus medius and gluteus maximus during rehabilitation exercises. Int J Sports Phys

Ther. 2011 Sep;6(3):206-23. PMID: 22034614; PMCID: PMC3201064.

38. Martín-Fuentes I, Oliva-Lozano JM, Muyor JM. Electromyographic activity in deadlift exercise and its variants. A systematic review. PLoS One. 2020 Feb 27;15(2):e0229507. doi: 10.1371/journal.pone.0229507. PMID: 32107499; PMCID: PMC

39. McAllister, M. J., Hammond, K. G., Schilling, B. K., Ferreria, L. C., Reed, J. P., & Weiss, L. W. (2014). Muscle activation during various hamstring exercises. Journal of Strength and Conditioning Research, 28(6), 1573-1580. https://doi.org/10.1519/JSC.0000000000000302

40. Mausehund, L., Skard, A. E., & Krosshaug, T. (2019). Muscle activation in unilateral barbell exercises: Implications for strength training and rehabilitation. Journal of Strength and Conditioning Research, 33(Suppl 1), S85-S94. https://doi.org/10.1519/JSC.0000000000002617

41. Gentil, P., Souza, D., Santana, M., Alves, R. R., Campos, M. H., Pinto, R., & Bottaro, M. (2020). Multi- and single-joint resistance exercises promote similar plantar flexor activation in

resistance trained men. International Journal of Environmental Research and Public Health, 17(24), 9487. https://doi.org/10.3390/ijerph17249487

42. Heidel, K. A., Novak, Z. J., & Dankel, S. J. (2022). Machines and free weight exercises: A systematic review and meta-analysis comparing changes in muscle size, strength, and power. Journal of Sports Medicine and Physical Fitness, 62(8), 1061-1070. https://doi.org/10.23736/S0022-4707.21.12929-9

43. Wilke, J., Stricker, V., & Usedly, S. (2020). Free-weight resistance exercise is more effective in enhancing inhibitory control than machine-based training: A randomized, controlled trial. Brain Sciences, 10(10), 702. https://doi.org/10.3390/brainsci10100702

44. Schwanbeck, S. R., Cornish, S. M., Barss, T., & Chilibeck, P. D. (2020). Effects of training with free weights versus machines on muscle mass, strength, free testosterone, and free cortisol levels. Journal of Strength and Conditioning Research, 34(7), 1851-1859. https://doi.org/10.1519/JSC.0000000000003349

45. Fischer SC, Calley DQ, Hollman JH. (2021). Effect of an exercise program that includes deadlifts on low back pain. Journal of Sport Rehabilitation, 30(4), 672-675. doi:10.1123/jsr.2020-0324

46. Curioni CC, Lourenço PM. (2005). Long-term weight loss after diet and exercise: A systematic review. International Journal of Obesity, 29(10), 1168-1174. doi:10.1038/sj.ijo.0803015

47. Lasikiewicz N, Myrissa K, Hoyland A, Lawton CL. (2014). Psychological benefits of weight loss following behavioural and/or dietary weight loss interventions: A systematic research review. Appetite, 72, 123-137. doi:10.1016/j.appet.2013.09.017

48. Lowry KW, Sallinen BJ, Janicke DM. (2007). The effects of weight management programs on self-esteem in pediatric overweight populations. Journal of Pediatric Psychology, 32(10), 1179-1195. doi:10.1093/jpepsy/jsm048

49. Martins, F. M., de Paula Souza, A., Nunes, P. R. P., Michelin, M. A., Murta, E. F. C., Resende, E. A. M. R., de Oliveira, E. P., & Orsatti, F. L. (2018). High-intensity body weight training is

comparable to combined training in changes in muscle mass, physical performance, inflammatory markers and metabolic health in postmenopausal women at high risk for type 2 diabetes mellitus: A randomized controlled clinical trial. Experimental Gerontology, 107, 108-115. doi:10.1016/j.exger.2018.02.016

50. Hall KD. What is the required energy deficit per unit weight loss? Int J Obes (Lond). 2008 Mar;32(3):573-6. doi: 10.1038/sj.ijo.0803720. Epub 2007 Sep 11. PMID: 17848938; PMCID: PMC2376744.

51. Zurlo F, Larson K, Bogardus C, Ravussin E. Skeletal muscle metabolism is a major determinant of resting energy expenditure. J Clin Invest. 1990 Nov;86(5):1423-7. doi: 10.1172/JCI114857. PMID: 2243122; PMCID: PMC296885.

52. ESPN. Retrieved from: https://www.espn.com/espn/story/_/id/27593253/why-grandmasters-magnus-carlsen-fabiano-caruana-lose-weight-playing-chess

53. Schott N, Johnen B, Holfelder B. Effects of free weights and machine training on muscular

strength in high-functioning older adults. Exp Gerontol. 2019 Jul 15;122:15-24. doi: 10.1016/j.exger.2019.03.012. Epub 2019 Apr 10. PMID: 30980922.

64